EAT LIKE A BOSS

Bodybuilding Meal Prep Cookbook And Guide For Females

Margaret T. Smith

Table of Contents

Chapter 1

What You Need To Build A Good Foundation That Guarantees Fantastic Results

The Macronutrient Needs Of Your Body And The Appropriate Ratios Of Protein, Carbohydrates, And Fats.

To fuel their rigorous workout regimens and develop lean muscle mass, female bodybuilders have special nutritional requirements. To achieve the best results and keep a healthy physique, one must be aware of the macronutrient needs of female bodybuilders. I will examine the macronutrient requirements of female physique builders in this session and offer advice for striking the right balance.

The nutrients that the body needs in substantial amounts to operate correctly are known as macronutrients. Protein, carbs, and fat are the three primary macronutrients. Each of these macronutrients has a specific function in the body and is necessary for preserving overall health, gaining muscle mass, and supplying energy.

The most crucial macronutrient for female bodybuilders is protein. It is required for keeping a strong immune system as well as for constructing and mending muscular tissue. The recommended daily protein intake for female bodybuilders is **1.2–1.7 grams** of protein per kilogram of body weight. This indicates that a lady weighing

120 pounds should try to eat 65 to 92 grams of protein per day.

Carbohydrates are also crucial since they give the body the energy it needs to power workouts. In the form of glycogen, which may be swiftly turned into energy during exercise, carbohydrates are stored in the muscles and liver. You should aim for **2-3 grams** of carbs per pound of body weight per day as a female bodybuilder. This indicates that if you are weighing 120 pounds, you should aim to eat 240 to 360 grams of carbs per day.

Fat is crucial for female bodybuilders as well since it gives the body the vital fatty acids that it cannot make on its own. The regulation of hormones and mental function both depend on fat. **0.5–1 gram** of fat per pound of body weight each day is the appropriate ratio for female bodybuilders. This indicates that if you are weighing 120 pounds, you should strive to eat between 60 and 120 grams of fat per day.

It's critical to balance all three macronutrients in each meal when designing a diet for bodybuilding. This will make it easier to make sure the body obtains the nutrition it needs to power workouts and develop muscle. Grilled chicken breast (protein), brown rice (carbohydrates), and mixed veggies sautéed in olive oil might make up a normal supper for a female bodybuilder (fat).

Overall, certain macronutrient requirements are needed for female bodybuilders to fuel their activities and develop lean muscle mass. A diet high in protein, carbs, and fat can assist in making sure your body has the resources it needs to maintain and develop muscle. You can obtain your ideal results and keep a healthy physique by understanding the macronutrient requirements of the body that has just been discussed and balancing the three macronutrients in your meals.

Having discussed the Macronutrient needs of your body as a female bodybuilder, it's expedient to strike a balance by exploring the micronutrient needs of your body as well.

The Micronutrient Requirements Of Female Body Builders And Advice For Striking The Right Balance

The body needs a little number of micronutrients, which include vitamins and minerals, to function effectively. Understanding the micronutrient requirements is just as crucial for female bodybuilders as understanding the macronutrient requirements. Micronutrients are essential for developing lean muscle mass, preserving general health, and avoiding disease.

The body's immune system, metabolism, bone health, and muscle function all depend on vitamins and minerals. For you to achieve your best results and retain excellent health as a bodybuilder, you must acquire adequate micronutrients. The following are some essential micronutrients that you need to know about:

Iron: Iron plays a crucial role in the delivery of oxygen to the muscles during exercise. Fatigue and poor performance during exercise are two effects of iron deficiency. Due to menstrual blood loss and a diet lacking in iron-rich foods, female bodybuilders are at risk for an iron shortage. Red meat, chicken, fish, beans, and dark leafy greens are among the foods rich in iron.

Calcium: Calcium is necessary for the development and maintenance of strong bones. Due to the demands of their training and diets low in calcium-rich foods, female bodybuilders are at risk for a calcium deficit. Dark leafy greens, fortified plant milk, and dairy products are some sources of calcium.

Vitamin D: Vitamin D is necessary for the absorption of calcium and the maintenance of healthy bones. Because of the demands of their training and limited sun exposure, female bodybuilders are at risk for vitamin D insufficiency. sources of vitamin D include fatty fish, fortified meals, and exposure to sunlight.

B vitamins: B vitamins are crucial for nerve and energy metabolism. Due to the demands of their training and a diet deficient in B vitamin-rich foods, female bodybuilders are at risk for B vitamin insufficiency. Lean meats, leafy greens, and whole grains are good sources of b vitamins.

Magnesium: Magnesium is necessary for the functioning of muscles and the creation of energy. Due to the demands of their training and diets low in magnesium-rich foods, female bodybuilders are at risk for magnesium shortage. Dark leafy greens, nuts, seeds, and whole grains are among the sources of magnesium.

You should focus on your overall food quality in addition to these micronutrients. Including a variety of fruits, vegetables, healthy grains, and lean protein sources in your diet will assist to ensure that you're getting all the micronutrients your body needs. For some people, supplementation may be necessary, but it's crucial to speak with a healthcare provider before beginning any supplementation program.

In summary, it is essential to comprehend the micronutrient requirements of female bodybuilders if you want to achieve the best results and keep yourself healthy. Among the essential micronutrients for you to be mindful of are iron, calcium, vitamin D, B vitamins, and magnesium. A diet centered on whole foods can aid in ensuring that your body receives all the essential micronutrients. You may make sure you are obtaining all the essential micronutrients to support your training and preserve good health by paying attention to the quality of your diet overall and talking to a healthcare practitioner.

How To Calculate And Track Calories And Macronutrients Intake

As a female bodybuilder, you need a well-balanced diet consisting of macronutrients (protein, carbs, and fats) and micronutrients (vitamins and minerals) to support your training and reach your fitness objectives. Calculating and monitoring calorie and macronutrient intake is vital for you to ensure that you are getting the proper quantity of nutrients for your demands. The following are the steps involved in calculating and monitoring calorie and macronutrient intake:

Step 1: Calculate Your Daily Caloric Requirements

The first step in estimating calorie and macronutrient intake is to establish your daily caloric requirements. This may be done using an internet calculator or by speaking with a trained dietician. Variables like age, height, weight, exercise level, and fitness objectives will all play a factor in establishing your daily calorie requirements.

Step 2: Establish Your Calorie And Macronutrient Objectives

After you have estimated your daily caloric requirements, the following step is to define your calorie and macronutrient targets. Depending on your objectives, you may want to strive for a certain ratio of macronutrients, such as a high-protein diet for muscle growth or a low-carb diet for weight reduction. Your calorie and macronutrient targets should be based on your specific requirements and should take into consideration your activity level and fitness objectives.

Step 3: Calculate And Monitor Your Calorie And Macronutrient Intake

The next step is to calculate and monitor your calorie and macronutrient consumption. There are various methods to achieve this, including:

1. **Using A Food Monitoring App:** There are numerous free applications available that enable you to track your calorie and macronutrient consumption by inputting the things you consume. These apps can also give you an overview of your nutrient intake and provide recommendations for meeting your goals.

2. **Keeping A Food Diary:** If you prefer to track your calorie and macronutrient intake manually, you can keep a food diary where you record the foods you eat and the

nutrient content of each food. This can be done using a spreadsheet or a notebook.

3. **Using A Kitchen Scale:** To effectively monitor your calorie and macronutrient consumption, you will need to measure your portions. Using a kitchen scale is an easy method to measure your meal quantities and verify that you are keeping within your calorie and macronutrient targets.

Step 4: Modify Your Intake As Required

After you have calculated and monitored your calorie and macronutrient consumption for a few weeks, you may need to change your intake depending on your results. If you are not experiencing the results you desire, you may need to modify your calorie and macronutrient intake to generate a greater deficit (if you are trying to lose weight) or a larger surplus (if you are attempting to develop muscle mass). On the other hand, if you are experiencing the results you desire, you may need to alter your intake to maintain your current weight or muscle mass.

To summarise, measuring and monitoring calorie and macronutrient consumption is vital for female bodybuilders who wish to attain their fitness objectives. By estimating your daily caloric requirements, setting calorie and macronutrient targets, and documenting your intake using a meal tracking app, food diary, or kitchen scale, you can guarantee that you are receiving the correct amount of nutrients to support your training and maintain excellent health. Speaking with a licensed dietician is always a smart idea to verify that individual requirements and objectives are being addressed.

Highly Recommended 10 Best Nutrition Apps To Use In Your Bodybuilding Journey

It's not always simple to eat healthily.

Yet, numerous apps with tools and information can help you achieve your nutritional objectives more quickly and easily than before.

I have compiled the 10 best nutrition apps to save you time. These applications are made to make eating healthier as simple as pressing a few buttons thanks to their favorable evaluations, top-notch content, and dependability.

1. The best nutrition app overall is MyPlate Calorie Counter.

2. PlateJoy is the top meal-planning app.
3. MyFitnessPal is the top meal-tracking app.

4. Yummly Recipes & Cooking Tools is the best app for healthy recipes.

5. The top app for losing weight is Lifesum: Healthy Eating

6. Ate Food Journal is the top app for mindful eating.

7. MyNet Diary Calorie Counter is the top macro counting app.

8. Noom is the top nutrition education app.

9. Spokin is the top food allergy app.

10.   Ovia Pregnancy Tracker is the best pregnancy nutrition app.

It's crucial to think about your objectives and the features that are most significant to you before choosing a nutrition app to download.

For instance, while some applications encourage mindful eating or nutrition education, others place a higher priority on calorie counting or weight loss.

Additionally, there are solutions designed expressly for persons who are expecting, have food allergies, or have unique nutritional needs or food preferences.

Choose apps that have received good reviews and endorsements from medical experts like doctors or nutritionists.

Take into account the app's usage fee as well. Certain apps may be available for free download and usage, however, there may be in-app membership fees or purchases available in other apps.

How Did I Select The Top Nutrition Apps?

Information quality: I searched for apps that provide trustworthy and beneficial dietary advice, especially from an authority figure like a qualified dietitian.

User interface: I searched for apps with simple user interfaces and clear navigation.

Nutritional requirements: I included apps that meet a range of nutritional requirements, from pregnancy and weight loss to meal planning and food tracking.

Customer reviews: To locate highly rated apps, I consulted with friends, family, and coworkers for recommendations and read through countless user reviews.

Apps have all been reviewed to make sure they adhere to Healthline's business and medical standards.

Chapter 2

Getting It Done With Supplements And Effective Meal Planning

Dietary Supplements And Their Function In Bodybuilding Nutrition

Bodybuilding is a form of exercise that focuses on developing and increasing muscle mass. While diet plays a vital role in building muscle, it can be challenging to get all the necessary nutrients from food alone. Dietary supplements are popular among bodybuilders, and they can play a crucial role in helping you achieve your goals. In this session, I will explore the role of dietary supplements in bodybuilding nutrition for female bodybuilders.

Protein Supplements

Protein is a vital nutrient for building and repairing muscles, and it is essential for bodybuilding. While protein can be found in foods such as meat, fish, eggs, and dairy, it can be difficult to consume enough protein through diet alone. This is where protein supplements can come in handy.

Protein is the most popular protein supplement for bodybuilders, as it is easily absorbed by the body and contains all the essential amino acids needed for muscle growth. Other protein supplements include casein protein, soy protein, and pea protein.

Amino Acids

Amino acids are the building blocks of protein, and they play a crucial role in building muscle. The body needs essential amino acids to synthesize muscle protein, and they cannot be produced by the body, which means they must be obtained from the diet or supplements.

Branch chain amino acids (BCAAs) are a popular supplement among bodybuilders since they are necessary amino acids that are digested directly in the muscle tissue. BCAAs may assist minimize muscle breakdown during exercise, increase muscular development, and aid in recuperation.

Creatine

Creatine is a natural substance found in the body and is also found in some foods. It is a popular supplement among bodybuilders, as it can help increase muscle mass, strength, and endurance.

Creatine works by providing the body with more energy during high-intensity exercise, allowing for more reps and sets. It can also help increase the water content in muscles, which can lead to a more significant increase in muscle size.

Beta-Alanine

Beta-alanine is an amino acid that is generated in the liver and is present in foods such as beef and fish. It is a popular supplement among bodybuilders, since it may assist boost muscular endurance and postpone muscle exhaustion.

Beta-alanine works by increasing the levels of carnosine in the muscles. Carnosine acts as a buffer, helping to reduce the build-up of lactic acid in the muscles during exercise, which can delay muscle fatigue.

Multivitamins

While a well-balanced diet can provide all the necessary vitamins and minerals needed for bodybuilding, it can be challenging to consume all the nutrients through food alone. Multivitamins can help ensure that the body is getting all the essential nutrients needed for muscle growth and repair.

Omega-3 Fatty Acids

Omega-3 fatty acids are essential fatty acids that cannot be produced by the body, meaning they must be obtained through diet or supplements. They are important for overall health and can also help reduce muscle inflammation and aid in muscle recovery.

Omega-3 supplements can be found in the form of fish oil or krill oil, and they can help reduce muscle soreness and inflammation after exercise.

In summary, nutritional supplements may play a key part in bodybuilding nutrition for female bodybuilders. Protein supplements, amino acids, creatine, beta-alanine, multivitamins, and omega-3 fatty acids may all assist boost muscle development, enhancing endurance, minimizing muscle fatigue, and aiding in muscle repair. Nevertheless, it is vital to note that supplements are not a substitute for a well-balanced diet, and they should be taken in combination with a healthy diet and exercise plan. It is also vital to contact a healthcare expert before beginning any supplement program.

Effective Meal Planning And Preparation Tips

Bodybuilding is a physically demanding activity that demands a well-planned diet to obtain the best results. Female bodybuilders need to pay additional attention to their food to gain lean muscle mass while maintaining a healthy weight. Meal planning and preparation will help you reach your fitness goals by ensuring you are obtaining the nutrients you need while also saving time and money. The following are some recommendations for food planning and preparation for you.

Prepare Your Meals Ahead of Time

The first step in good meal planning and preparation is to schedule your meals ahead of time. Spend some time each week to plan out your meals for the next week. Start by picking your protein sources, such as chicken, fish, or tofu, and then put in your carbs, such as sweet potatoes, brown rice, or quinoa. Lastly, toss in some healthy fats, such as avocado, almonds, or seeds. Be sure to incorporate a variety of veggies and fruits as well.

Prep Your Ingredients in Advance

After you have your meal plan for the week, you can start preparing your supplies in advance. Chop up your veggies, marinate your meats, and prepare your grains in advance, so they are ready to use when you need them. This will save you time throughout the week when you are busy with work and training.

Invest in Meal Prep Containers

Investing in meal prep containers is a wonderful way to keep organized and ensure that you have nutritious meals on hand throughout the week. Look for containers that are microwave and dishwasher-safe, as well as leak-proof, so you can take them with you on the go.

Cook in Bulk

Cooking in bulk is another fantastic method to save time and money while ensuring you have nutritious meals on hand. Select a day of the week to prepare a big quantity of your protein and carbohydrate sources, such as chicken and brown rice, and then divide them out into your meal prep containers. You may also create huge amounts of soups or stews that can be refrigerated and warmed later in the week.

Employ Herbs and Spices to Add Flavor

With meal planning and preparation, it is necessary to consider taste as well. Dull meals may be uninteresting and lead to the desire for unhealthy foods. Herbs and spices may add flavor to your meals without adding additional calories or salt. Experiment with various herbs and spices to discover combinations that you prefer.

Integrate Snacks into Your Meal Plan

Snacks are a vital element of any diet plan, particularly for female bodybuilders who need to ingest enough calories to power their exercises. Healthy snack alternatives include fruit, almonds, yogurt, or hummus with veggies.

In summary, Meal planning and preparation are essential for female bodybuilders looking to achieve their fitness goals. By planning your meals ahead of time, prepping your ingredients in advance, investing in meal prep containers, cooking in bulk, using herbs and spices to add flavor, and incorporating snacks into your meal plan, you can save time, and money, and ensure that you are getting the nutrients you need to build lean muscle mass and maintain a healthy weight.

Food Shopping Tactics

As a female bodybuilder, you are likely to have special nutritional needs that vary from those of a normal individual. Grocery shopping may be a difficult process, particularly if you are not aware of what to look for. Nevertheless, with a few basic tactics, you can make your shopping trip quicker and more effective while still ensuring that you are achieving your nutritional requirements.

Plan Ahead

Before you travel to the grocery store, take some time to plan your meals for the week. This will allow you to identify what items you need to purchase and ensure that you have everything on hand to produce healthy and balanced meals. Try drafting a shopping list to keep you on track and eliminate impulsive purchases.

Shop The Perimeter Of The Shop

As you enter the grocery store, you may notice that the fresh vegetables, meats, and dairy items are positioned around the perimeter of the shop. This is because these things are often less processed and more nutrient-dense than the packaged and processed foods that are available in the aisles. Make it a point to spend most of your time in these places to ensure that you are obtaining the nutrients that your body requires.

Seek For High-protein Meals

As a bodybuilder, protein is necessary for growing and repairing muscle tissue. Seek high-protein foods such as lean meats, fish, eggs, and low-fat dairy items. Plant-based protein sources such as legumes, nuts, and seeds are also excellent choices. Consider purchasing protein powder to supplement your diet if you are struggling to get enough protein from food alone.

Choose Healthy Fats

Healthy fats are important for maintaining optimal health and performance. Look for sources of healthy fats such as avocados, nuts, seeds, and olive oil, and fatty fish such as salmon. Avoid processed and fried meals that are rich in harmful fats.

Don't Forget About Carbohydrates

While protein is essential for building and repairing muscle, carbohydrates are important for providing the energy your body needs to power through your workouts. Choose complex carbohydrates such as whole grains, fruits, and vegetables, rather than simple carbohydrates found in processed and sugary foods.

Read Food Labels

When shopping for packaged and processed foods, it's important to read the nutrition labels. Look for foods that are low in sugar and saturated fat, and high in fiber and protein. Be wary of marketing claims such as "low fat" or "low sugar," as these foods may be highly processed and contain other unhealthy ingredients.

Consider Buying In Bulk

Buying in bulk can save you money and ensure that you have a steady supply of healthy foods on hand. Try buying products such as rice, oats, and almonds in quantity. You may also buy frozen fruits and veggies in quantity, which can be a handy and cost-effective choice.

In summary, grocery shopping as a female bodybuilder may be a tough but gratifying experience. By planning, shopping the perimeter of the store, and picking nutritious, nutrient-dense foods, you can guarantee that you are fulfilling your nutritional requirements and feeding your body for maximum performance.

Chapter 3

Sources And Recipes

Protein-rich Food Sources

Protein is an important component that plays a crucial part in the development and repair of our bodily structures. It is also needed for the creation of enzymes, hormones, and other bodily components. Our body cannot store protein, thus we need to ingest it consistently via our food. In this session, I will examine some of the greatest sources of protein-rich foods that you may integrate into your diet.

Beef and Poultry: Beef and poultry are great sources of high-quality protein, which is important for muscle development and repair. Chicken, turkey, beef, and pork are some of the most common varieties of meat that are rich in protein. A 3-ounce amount of cooked chicken breast offers around 26 grams of protein, whereas a 3-ounce dish of beef contains about 22 grams of protein.

Seafood: Seafood is also a good source of protein and other critical elements. Fish such as salmon, tuna, and sardines are rich in protein and omega-3 fatty acids, which are helpful for heart health. A 3-ounce portion of grilled salmon offers around 22 grams of protein, whereas a 3-ounce serving of canned tuna contains about 20 grams of protein.

Eggs: Eggs are an excellent source of protein, and they are also flexible and quick to cook. One big egg offers around 6 grams of protein, and it may be cooked, scrambled, or turned into an omelet. Egg whites are also a good source of protein and are regularly used by athletes and bodybuilders to increase their protein intake.

Dairy Products: Dairy products such as milk, cheese, and yogurt are also rich sources of protein. Greek yogurt is especially rich in protein, with a 6-ounce serving has roughly 17 grams of protein. Low-fat cottage cheese is also a fantastic source of protein, with a half-cup serving has roughly 14 grams of protein.

Nuts and Seeds: Nuts and seeds are a terrific source of plant-based protein, and they also include healthy fats and other critical components. Almonds, peanuts, and pistachios are some of the most common varieties of nuts that are rich in protein. A quarter-cup serving of almonds contains about 7 grams of protein, while a quarter-cup serving of pumpkin seeds contains about 9 grams of protein.

Legumes: Legumes such as lentils, beans, and chickpeas are also excellent sources of protein, and they are often used as vegetarian or vegan protein sources. A half-cup serving of cooked lentils contains about 9 grams of protein, while a half-cup serving of cooked black beans contains about 8 grams of protein.

To conclude This session, there are many sources of protein-rich foods that you can incorporate into your diet. Whether you favor meat, fish, dairy products, nuts, seeds, or legumes, there are lots of alternatives to select from. By integrating these protein-rich foods into your meals, you can guarantee that you are achieving your daily protein needs and supporting your overall health and well-being.

How To Prepare Protein-rich Foods In Various Ways

Grilling or Roasting Meat and Poultry

Grilling or roasting meat and poultry is a great way to prepare protein-rich foods. Chicken breasts, turkey, beef, and pork are excellent sources of high-quality protein. Grilling or roasting these meats improves their natural taste and helps to maintain their nutrients. For optimal results, marinade the meat or poultry with your preferred spices, herbs, and a small amount of oil before grilling or roasting.

Steaming or Boiling Seafood

Seafood is another fantastic source of protein, and it is simple to prepare by steaming or boiling. Fish such as salmon, trout, and tuna are rich in omega-3 fatty acids and protein. To make steamed fish, put the fish in a steamer basket and cook for 10-15 minutes. Boiling seafood such as shrimp or crab is also a wonderful technique to cook them. To boil shrimp, bring a saucepan of water to a boil, add the shrimp, and simmer for 2-3 minutes until they become pink.

Baking Eggs

Eggs are a flexible protein source that may be cooked in numerous ways. One of the simplest methods to cook eggs is by baking them. Preheat the oven to 350°F, break the eggs into a greased baking dish, season with salt and pepper, and bake for 15-20 minutes. Cooked eggs may be eaten with whole-grain bread or blended with veggies for a delightful breakfast or brunch.

Using Greek Yogurt in Recipes

Greek yogurt is a good source of protein and may be used in numerous dishes. It is an excellent alternative to sour cream or mayonnaise and may be used in dips, salads, and sauces. Greek yogurt may also be used to create smoothies, parfaits, and even desserts. Mixing some fruit and nuts with Greek yogurt provides a delightful and healthful snack.

Adding Legumes to Salads and Soups

Legumes such as lentils, beans, and chickpeas are excellent sources of plant-based protein. They may be added to salads, soups, and stews for a protein boost. To create lentil salad, simmer the lentils in water until cooked, and then combine them with chopped veggies and a vinaigrette dressing. For a protein-rich soup, simmer a blend of beans and veggies in broth until soft and season with your preferred seasonings.

In conclusion, there are various methods to cook protein-rich meals to maintain a balanced diet. Whether you prefer meat, seafood, eggs, Greek yogurt, or legumes, there are plenty of options to choose from. By integrating these protein-rich foods into your meals, you can guarantee that you are achieving your daily protein needs and supporting your overall health and well-being.

How To Include Protein-rich Foods into Your Meals

Including protein-rich foods in your meals is vital for maintaining a healthy and balanced diet. Protein is needed for creating and repairing tissues, supporting a strong immune system, and keeping healthy bones and muscles. It also helps keep you feeling full and satisfied, which may avoid overeating and improve weight reduction.

The following are how to add protein-rich foods to your meals.

Start with Breakfast

Breakfast is a fantastic opportunity to integrate protein-rich items into your meals. Eggs, Greek yogurt, and protein smoothies are all fantastic alternatives. You may also add protein to your breakfast by including protein-rich items like nuts, seeds, or nut butter in your oatmeal or smoothie.

Prepare High-Protein Snacks

Snacks are a fantastic chance to integrate protein-rich foods into your diet. Hard-boiled eggs, roasted chickpeas, and almonds are all healthful and protein-packed snack alternatives. You may also prepare a protein-rich dip by combining Greek yogurt with spices and herbs, or hummus with vegetables.

Add Protein to Your Salads

Adding protein to your salad is a simple method to enhance your protein consumption. Grilled chicken, fish, tofu, or beans are all wonderful protein options that may be added to a salad. You may also add nuts, seeds, or cheese for added protein and texture.

Select Protein-rich Side Dishes

Incorporate protein-rich side dishes into your meals, such as roasted or grilled veggies, baked sweet potatoes, or quinoa salad. These sides are a fantastic way to add nutrition and protein to your meal.

Choose Lean Protein Sources

When picking protein sources, it's crucial to select lean choices. Some wonderful lean protein sources are chicken breast, turkey breast, seafood, beans, and lentils. Lean protein sources are lower in calories and fat, making them a healthier alternative.

Integrate Protein into Your Desserts

Believe it or not, it's easy to add protein to your sweets. Greek yogurt, protein powder, or cottage cheese may be utilized to generate protein-packed dessert alternatives such as protein pudding, protein bars, or protein smoothies.

In conclusion, integrating protein-rich foods into your meals is vital for maintaining a healthy and balanced diet. By beginning with breakfast, producing high-protein snacks, adding protein to your salads and side dishes, selecting lean protein sources, and including protein in your sweets, you can easily improve your protein consumption and support your overall health and well-being. Remember to always pick complete, nutrient-dense meals that feed your body and give the protein it needs.

Healthy carbohydrate sources and how to include them in meals

Carbohydrates are an important macronutrient that supplies energy to our bodies. Nevertheless, not all carbohydrate sources are created equal. Certain carbs, such as processed sugars and white wheat, may contribute to blood sugar increases and weight gain. On the other side, nutritious carbohydrate sources including whole grains, fruits, and vegetables give critical vitamins, minerals, and fiber. Below are healthy carbohydrate sources and how to include them in meals.

Whole Grains

Whole grains are a fantastic source of nutritious carbs. They are rich in fiber, vitamins, and minerals, and may help lessen the risk of heart disease, type 2 diabetes, and some malignancies. Examples of entire grains include brown rice, quinoa, oats, and whole-grain bread. To integrate whole grains into your meals, consider substituting white rice with brown rice, preparing a quinoa salad, or using whole-grain bread for sandwiches.

Fruits

Fruits are a nutritious source of carbs that are also filled with critical vitamins and minerals. They may be eaten fresh or cooked and are a terrific way to satisfy your sweet taste. Examples of fruits that are rich in healthy carbohydrates include bananas, apples, oranges, and berries. To incorporate fruit into your meals, try adding berries to your oatmeal, making a fruit smoothie, or topping your pancakes with sliced bananas.

Vegetables

Vegetables are an excellent source of healthy carbohydrates that are also low in calories.

They are rich in fiber, vitamins, and minerals and can help lower the risk of heart disease, type 2 diabetes, and certain cancers. Examples of vegetables that are rich in healthy carbohydrates include sweet potatoes, peas, corn, and leafy greens. To incorporate vegetables into your meals, try making a roasted vegetable medley, adding leafy greens to your salad, or using sweet potatoes instead of white potatoes.

Legumes

Legumes are a healthy source of carbohydrates that are also high in protein and fiber. They can help lower the risk of heart disease, type 2 diabetes, and certain cancers. Examples of legumes that are rich in healthy carbohydrates include lentils, chickpeas, black beans, and kidney beans. To incorporate legumes into your meals, try making a lentil soup, adding black beans to your salad, or making a chickpea curry.

Dairy

Dairy products like milk and yogurt are a healthy source of carbohydrates that are also rich in calcium and vitamin D. These may help maintain strong bones and teeth. To integrate dairy into your meals, consider adding yogurt to your smoothie, preparing a yogurt parfait with fruit and granola, or using milk in your oatmeal.

In summary, nutritious carbohydrate sources are necessary for keeping a healthy and balanced diet. Whole grains, fruits, vegetables, legumes, and dairy products are all wonderful sources of nutritious carbs that may be included in meals in several ways. Remember to pick full, nutrient-dense meals that fuel your body and offer the energy it needs to flourish

Healthy Fat Sources And How To Include Them Into Meals

Fat is an essential macronutrient that plays a critical role in maintaining overall health. It helps our body absorb certain vitamins, promotes cognitive function, and offers energy. However, not all fats are created equal. Good fats are important for optimum health, but bad fats may lead to weight gain and raise the risk of heart disease. Below are the healthy fat sources and how to include them in meals.

Avocado

Avocado is a healthy source of monounsaturated and polyunsaturated fats, which may help decrease cholesterol levels and reduce the risk of heart disease. It is also an excellent source of fiber, potassium, and vitamins C and K. To include avocado in your meals, consider adding it to your salad, preparing guacamole, or using it as a spread on your sandwich.

Nuts and Seeds

Nuts and seeds are a nutritious source of polyunsaturated and monounsaturated fats, fiber, and protein. They may help decrease inflammation and minimize the risk of heart disease. Examples of nuts and seeds that are high in healthful fats include almonds, walnuts, chia seeds, and flax seeds. To integrate nuts and seeds into your meals, consider adding them to your oatmeal, preparing a trail mix, or using them as a topping for your salad.

Fatty Fish

Fatty fish like salmon, tuna, and mackerel are excellent sources of omega-3 fatty acids, which can help reduce inflammation and lower the risk of heart disease. They are also a good source of protein and vitamin D. To incorporate fatty fish into your meals, try making grilled salmon, tuna salad, or adding canned salmon to your pasta.

Olive Oil

Olive oil is a healthy source of monounsaturated fats, which can help lower cholesterol levels and reduce the risk of heart disease. It is also rich in antioxidants, which may help decrease inflammation. To include olive oil in your meals, consider using it as a dressing for your salad, sautéing your veggies, or spreading it over your spaghetti.

Coconut

Coconut is a healthy source of medium-chain triglycerides, which are a type of saturated fat that can help boost energy levels and reduce inflammation. It is also rich in fiber and antioxidants. To incorporate coconut into your meals, try adding shredded coconut to your oatmeal, making coconut milk-based curry, or using coconut oil to bake your favorite treats.

In conclusion, healthy fat sources are essential for maintaining overall health. Avocado, nuts and seeds, fatty fish, olive oil, and coconut are all excellent sources of healthy fats that can be incorporated into meals in a variety of ways. Remember to choose healthy fats in moderation and pair them with other nutrient-dense foods to create balanced and delicious meals.

Ideas For High-protein Meals And Snacks That Are Particularly Developed For Female Bodybuilders

Female bodybuilders have special dietary demands that are distinct from those of male bodybuilders. Women require a larger amount of protein in their diet to promote muscle development and repair. In this session, I will examine ideas for high-protein meals and snacks that are particularly developed for female bodybuilders.

High-Protein Breakfast: Greek Yogurt Bowl

Greek yogurt is a wonderful source of protein and calcium. To create this high-protein breakfast, combine 1 cup of plain Greek yogurt with 1/2 cup of mixed berries and top with 2 tablespoons of chopped almonds. This breakfast is filled with protein, fiber, and healthy fats, making it the ideal start to a busy day.

High-Protein Snack: Edamame

Edamame is a terrific high-protein snack that is suitable for female bodybuilders. To create this snack, boil 1 cup of edamame in salted water for 5 minutes. Drain and sprinkle with sea salt. Edamame is a good source of plant-based protein and fiber, making it a terrific snack to fuel your exercise.

High-Protein Lunch: Grilled Chicken Salad

Grilled chicken salad is a traditional high-protein dish that is great for female bodybuilders. To create this salad, grill 4 ounces of chicken breast and slice it into strips. Toss 2 cups of mixed greens with 1/2 cup of chopped veggies of your choice and top with the sliced chicken. Drizzle with a homemade vinaigrette made with 2 tablespoons of olive oil and 1 tablespoon of apple cider vinegar. This meal is packed with protein, fiber, and healthy fats, making it the perfect lunch to fuel your workouts.

High-Protein Snack: Peanut Butter Apple Slices

Peanut butter apple slices are a great high-protein snack that is perfect for female bodybuilders. To make this snack, slice 1 apple into thin slices and spread with 2 tablespoons of peanut butter. Sprinkle with cinnamon and a drizzle of honey. Peanut butter is an excellent source of protein and healthy fats, making it a great snack to fuel your workouts.

High-Protein Dinner: Salmon Quinoa Bowl

The salmon quinoa bowl is a high-protein meal that is perfect for female bodybuilders. To make this meal, cook 1 cup of quinoa according to the package instructions. Grill 4 ounces of salmon and flake into small pieces. Toss the quinoa with 1/2 cup of mixed veggies of your choice and top with the grilled salmon. Drizzle with a homemade vinaigrette made with 2 tablespoons of olive oil and 1 tablespoon of lemon juice. This meal is packed with protein, fiber, and healthy fats, making it the perfect dinner to fuel your workouts.

In conclusion, female bodybuilders have distinct nutritional demands that need a larger amount of protein in their diet. These recipes for high-protein meals and snacks are particularly intended to help muscle development and repair. Adding these dishes to your diet will help you reach your fitness goals and fuel your exercises.

Chapter 4

Workout and Meal Timing Strategies

Strategies For Fueling Workouts And Maximizing Recovery

When it comes to accomplishing your fitness objectives, feeding your efforts and boosting recuperation are just as crucial as the actual activities you undertake. A good diet may assist increase performance, minimizing tiredness, and promoting recovery, enabling you to get the most out of your exercises. In this session, I will examine tactics for fuelling workouts and boosting recuperation.

Hydration

One of the most essential things you can do to fuel your workouts and encourage recovery is to keep hydrated. Dehydration may lead to tiredness, poor performance, and delayed recovery. Try to drink water throughout the day, and be sure you drink enough water before, during, and after your exercise.

Pre-Workout Nutrition

Consuming the correct meals before a workout will assist supply your body with the energy it needs to function at its best. Concentrate on consuming complex carbs, such as fruits, vegetables, and whole grains, which give continuous energy throughout your exercise. Also, ingesting protein before an exercise might aid minimize muscle breakdown and boost recovery. Try consuming a modest lunch or snack 30 minutes to an hour before your exercise.

During-Workout Nutrition

If your exercise is longer than 60 minutes, try ingesting carbs throughout your workout to assist sustain energy levels. Sports drinks or gels may be a good source of quickly-digested carbs.

Post-Workout Nutrition

Following an exercise, it's vital to ingest protein and carbs to enhance recuperation and restore energy reserves. Concentrate on having a meal or snack within 30 minutes after completing your exercise to encourage maximum recovery. Items such as lean protein sources, like chicken or fish, and complex carbs, such as sweet potatoes or quinoa, may be terrific selections.

Rest and Recovery

Adequate rest and recuperation are vital for optimizing the advantages of your exercises. Give your body time to relax and recuperate between exercises, and be sure you get enough sleep each night. Strive for 7-9 hours of sleep each night to support healthy recovery and prevent weariness.

In conclusion, feeding your exercises and optimizing recuperation is crucial for attaining your fitness objectives. By remaining hydrated, taking the necessary nutrients before, during, and after your exercise, and giving your body sufficient rest and recovery time, you may optimize the advantages of your workouts and reach your fitness objectives. Talk with a healthcare physician or certified dietitian for individualized dietary recommendations based on your unique requirements and objectives.

Meal Timing Strategies For Pre And Post-workout Nutrition

When it comes to working out, fuelling your body correctly is vital for maximum performance and recovery. Pre- and post-exercise meals are key components of any fitness regimen, supplying the energy and nutrition required to power through a workout and help the body recuperate afterward.

Pre-Workout Food Ideas

Oatmeal: A cup of oatmeal is an excellent source of complex carbs, giving long-lasting energy for your exercise. Add some nuts or berries for added nutrition and taste.

Banana: A simple banana delivers quick-digesting carbs and potassium, which helps avoid muscular cramping throughout your exercise.

Greek yogurt: Rich in protein and low in sugar, Greek yogurt is a terrific pre-workout snack. Add some fruit or granola for added carbs.

Smoothie: Mix a smoothie with fruit, Greek yogurt, and some protein powder for a fast and simple pre-workout meal. It's a fantastic source of carbs, protein, and electrolytes.

Whole-grain toast with peanut butter: A piece of whole-grain bread covered with peanut butter is a wonderful mix of protein, healthy fats, and carbs, ideal for supplying energy before your exercise.

Post-Workout Lunch Ideas

Grilled chicken with veggies: Grilled chicken is a fantastic source of protein, while vegetables give vitamins and minerals required for muscle repair. Add some quinoa or brown rice for additional carbs.

Smoothie bowl: Blend up a smoothie with some fruit and Greek yogurt, and top it with granola, nuts, and seeds for an excellent source of carbohydrates, protein, and healthy fats.

Baked sweet potato: Sweet potatoes are high in complex carbohydrates, fiber, and vitamins. Top with some Greek yogurt and cinnamon for a satisfying post-workout meal.

Tuna or salmon with quinoa and vegetables: Tuna and salmon are high in protein and omega-3 fatty acids, which are essential for muscle recovery. Add some quinoa and veggies for added nutrients and carbs.

Chocolate milk: Chocolate milk is a great post-workout drink, providing carbohydrates and protein to replenish energy stores and promote muscle recovery.

All in all, Pre- and post-workout meals are essential components of any fitness routine, providing the energy and nutrients needed to power through a workout and help the body recover afterward. Integrating these meal ideas into your routine will help increase performance, promote recovery, and support overall health and well-being. Remember to listen to your body and alter your meals appropriately, depending on your specific requirements and tastes.

Meal Timing Strategies For Pre And Post-workout Nutrition

When it comes to nutrition for exercise, mealtime is a vital aspect. Appropriate meal timing may assist maximize performance during an exercise, stimulate muscle repair and development, and boost overall health and well-being. In this session, I'll discuss several Meal timing strategies for pre- and post-workout nutrition

Pre-Workout Food Timing Strategies

Scheduling your pre-exercise breakfast is vital to ensuring that your body has enough energy to get through your workout. Preferably, you should consume a meal or snack 30 minutes to 3 hours before your exercise. Here are some strategies to consider:

1. **Take a light lunch or snack 30 minutes to 1 hour before your workout:** If you're short on time, having a little breakfast or snack shortly before your exercise might give you a rapid dose of energy. Select meals that are simple to digest and low in fat, protein, and fiber, such as a banana, apple slices with nut butter, or a smoothie.

2. **Have a bigger supper 2-3 hours before your workout:** If you have more time before your activity, a bigger lunch might give you continuous energy for your workout. Select meals that are rich in complex carbs, such as whole grains, sweet potatoes, or quinoa, as well as some lean protein and healthy fats.

3. **Experiment with meal time:** Everyone's body is different, so it's vital to experiment with meal timing

to determine what works best for you. Some individuals may find that they do better with a bigger lunch a few hours before their exercise, while others may prefer a smaller snack shortly before their activity.

Post-Workout Food Timing Strategies

Timing your post-workout meal is critical to optimize muscle repair and development. Preferably, you should consume a meal or snack between 30 minutes to 2 hours following your exercise. Here are some strategies to consider:

1. **Eat a meal or snack immediately after your workout:** After your workout, your body is in a state of heightened nutrient uptake, so it's important to provide it with the nutrients it needs. Choose foods that are high in carbohydrates and protein,

such as a smoothie with protein powder, a sandwich with turkey and avocado, or Greek yogurt with fruit.

2. **Eat a larger meal within 2 hours after your workout:** If you have more time after your workout, a larger meal can help promote muscle recovery and growth. Choose foods that are high in complex carbohydrates, lean protein, and healthy fats, such as grilled chicken with vegetables and quinoa, or a salmon salad with avocado and nuts.

3. **Consider nutrient timing:** In addition to meal timing, nutrient timing can also be important for post-workout nutrition. For example, consuming carbohydrates immediately after your workout can help replenish glycogen stores, while consuming protein can help promote muscle recovery and growth.

In summary, Proper meal timing is important for pre- and post-workout nutrition. By scheduling your meals and snacks carefully, you can supply your body with the energy and nutrition it needs to push through your exercise and encourage muscle repair and development. Remember to experiment with various meal scheduling techniques to discover what works best for you, and to emphasize nutrient-dense meals that promote overall health and well-being.

Chapter 5

Workable Methods

Workable Methods For Eating Out And Sticking To A Bodybuilding Meal Plan When Traveling

Traveling might provide a problem when it comes to keeping to a bodybuilding eating plan. Dining out at restaurants may be appealing, with infinite selections and the ease of not having to prepare meals. Yet, with a few suggestions and methods, it is feasible to eat out while still keeping to your bodybuilding diet plan. The following are workable methods for eating out and adhering to a bodybuilding diet plan while traveling.

1. **Prepare Ahead:** Before your vacation, do some research and identify eateries that provide healthy selections. Several restaurants now feature menus that cater to particular dietary demands, including low-carb, high-protein, and gluten-free alternatives. Search for eateries that provide grilled or baked meats, veggies, and healthful grains.

2. **Be Prepared:** If you know you'll be on the run for a long period, carry food with you. Bring protein bars, almonds, and dried fruit for a fast and simple snack on the move. This may help keep you from reaching for harmful choices when hunger hits.

3. **Make Modifications:** Don't be scared to ask for alterations to your

food. Ask for grilled or baked meats, additional veggies, and nutritious grains instead of processed carbs. Most restaurants are willing to make replacements and alterations to satisfy dietary preferences.

4. **Practice Portion Control:** Restaurant servings are generally significantly greater than what you would cook at home. Try sharing lunch with a buddy or taking half of your meal to go for later. This might help you avoid overeating and remain inside your bodybuilding food plan.

5. **Be Aware of Your Choices:** Be conscious of the choices you make while dining out. Avoid fried meals, thick sauces, and large quantities of cheese or butter. Select grilled, baked, or steamed meats and vegetables, and choose healthy fats like avocado or olive oil.

6. **Adhere to Your Macros:** If you are monitoring your macros, make careful to keep to them while dining out. Search for meals that fall within your macro objectives, and alter your quantities and selections appropriately.

7. **Don't Forget About Hydration:** Keeping hydrated is vital for general health and well-being, and may also help you remain on track with your bodybuilding food plan. Drink lots of water throughout the day, and avoid sugary beverages like soda or juice.

Dining out while keeping to a bodybuilding meal plan may be a problem, but with a little forethought and preparation, it is feasible to make nutritious choices while on the run. By exercising portion control, making adaptations, and being conscious of your choices, you may enjoy eating out while being on track with your bodybuilding objectives. Remember to emphasize nutrient-dense meals that promote overall health and well-being, and to remain hydrated during your trips

Workable Methods For Adhering To A Bodybuilding Food Plan While Eating With Friends

Adhering to a bodybuilding food plan may be tough, particularly when eating out with companions who may not share your nutritional objectives. It might be tempting to indulge in unhealthy foods or skip meals completely, but with a little forethought and attention, it is easy to remain on track with your bodybuilding diet plan while still enjoying time with friends. In this part, I will cover some methods for adhering to a bodybuilding food plan while eating with friends.

1. **Prepare Ahead:** Before heading out to eat, check the restaurant's menu online and pick healthy alternatives that fit within your bodybuilding meal plan. Many restaurants now offer low-carb, high-protein, and gluten-free options that can be easily

customized to meet your dietary needs. By planning ahead, you can avoid making impulsive, unhealthy choices when you arrive at the restaurant.

2. **Communicate with Your Friends:** Let your friends know about your bodybuilding goals and the importance of sticking to your meal plan. This can help them understand why you may not be indulging in certain foods and can also help them support you in your efforts.

3. **Don't Be Afraid to Make Modifications:** Many restaurants are happy to accommodate dietary needs and make modifications to dishes. Don't be hesitant to ask for grilled or baked meats, additional veggies, and nutritious grains instead of processed carbs. By making modifications, you can ensure that

your meal fits within your bodybuilding meal plan.

4. **Practice Portion Control:** Restaurant servings are generally significantly greater than what you would cook at home. Try sharing lunch with a buddy or taking half of your meal to go for later. This might help you avoid overeating and remain inside your bodybuilding food plan.

5. **Be Mindful of Your Choices:** When dining out, be mindful of your choices. Avoid fried meals, thick sauces, and large quantities of cheese or butter. Select grilled, baked, or steamed meats and vegetables, and choose healthy fats like avocado or olive oil.

6. **Don't Skip Meals:** It can be tempting to skip meals when dining out with friends, especially if there

aren't many healthy options available. Yet, missing meals may lead to overeating later on and can also damage your general energy levels. Instead, eat smaller, nutrient-dense meals throughout the day to keep on track with your bodybuilding meal plan.

7. **Appreciate the Company:** Although keeping to a bodybuilding diet plan is crucial, it is equally important to enjoy the company of your friends. Concentrate on the social component of eating out, rather than merely on the cuisine. Remember that a single meal won't make or break your bodybuilding ambitions and that it's alright to eat in moderation.

Adhering to a bodybuilding diet plan while eating with friends may be tough, but with a little forethought and attention, it is easy to remain on track while still enjoying time with loved ones. By planning ahead, communicating with your friends, making modifications, practicing portion control, being mindful of your choices, not skipping meals, and focusing on the social aspect of dining out, you can stay on track with your bodybuilding goals and also have a great time with your friends. Remember that consistency is key, and that small, healthy choices over time can lead to significant progress toward your bodybuilding goals.

Chapter 6

Ultimate Pieces Of Advice

Advice For Managing Cravings

Many people frequently feel cravings. Cravings can be challenging to control, whether they are a sudden yearning for a certain meal or a strong desire to partake in a particular activity. Yet you can manage your urges and stop them from harming your health and well-being if you take the appropriate approach.

Recognize The Root Cause

Finding the source of the urge is one of the most crucial steps in managing it. Cravings frequently result from an emotional or physical desire. For instance, you might seek comfort food if you're stressed or anxious to relax. As an alternative, your body may tell your brain that you are hungry if you are dehydrated or haven't eaten in a while.

You can take action to immediately treat your craving's underlying source once you've determined what it is. Consider doing something calming like yoga or meditation if you're feeling anxious. Make sure to have a balanced dinner or snack if you're hungry.

Keep Hydrated

Staying hydrated throughout the day is vital because cravings can be brought on by dehydration. Water might make you feel satiated and lessen the severity of your cravings. If you're physically engaged or in a hot setting, aim to consume at least eight glasses of water each day.

Become Distracted

When a need strikes, it can be beneficial to divert your attention to something that demands your complete focus. This can assist divert your attention from the urge and lessen how strong it is. Consider taking a stroll, reading a book, or doing a puzzle.

Adopt a Mindful Eating Habit

Mindful eating involves focusing on the flavor, texture, and aroma of the food. Spend some time enjoying each meal rather than eating quickly. This can increase your eating enjoyment and lessen your propensity to overeat. It's also vital to eat slowly because it takes your brain about 20 minutes to realize that you are full.

Think Ahead

Plan ahead if you are aware of a specific craving you may have. For instance, instead of fully depriving yourself if you're desiring chocolate, make plans to eat a tiny amount after dinner. This can assist you in giving in to your urge without going overboard.

Obtain Enough Sleep

It's crucial to get enough rest because getting too little sleep might make desires worse. To aid your body's natural cycles, aim for seven to eight hours of sleep each night and create a reliable sleep regimen.

Locate Better Alternatives

Try to find a healthier substitute if you are seeking anything sweet or salty. For instance, if you're in the mood for ice cream, consider freezing some fruit and making sorbet out of it. Instead of reaching for chips when you're hungry, try some roasted nuts or vegetables.

Although cravings are a normal aspect of life, they don't have to rule your life. You can healthily control your desires and enhance your general health and well-being by comprehending the source of your cravings, staying hydrated, choosing healthier substitutes, practicing mindful eating, planning, getting adequate sleep, and engaging in distraction techniques.

Advice For Managing Binge Eating

A widespread problem that impacts many people is binge eating. It is described as eating a lot of food in a short amount of time while frequently experiencing remorse or embarrassment. Obesity, diabetes, and melancholy are just a few of the devastating effects that binge eating may have on one's physical and mental well-being. You may take measures to prevent binge eating and keep a positive connection with food, though.

Recognize Your Triggers

To prevent binge eating, one of the most crucial tasks is to become aware of your triggers. Triggers are events or feelings that make you eat in a harmful way. A few typical causes are tension, fear, boredom, and depressive thoughts. When you know what your triggers are, you can either avoid them or healthily deal with them.

Adopt a Mindful Eating Habit

Mindful eating involves focusing on the flavor, texture, and aroma of the food. Also, it entails chewing each bite thoroughly and gently. When you eat mindfully, you become more conscious of when you are full, which can prevent overeating. You are also more likely to enjoy your food, which can aid in avoiding emotions of deprivation that might trigger binge eating.

Eat Typical Meals

Binge eating can result from skipping meals. Your body could become extremely hungry if you skip meals, which could lead to overeating when you do eat. Make sure to consume regular meals throughout the day to prevent this. Try to eat three meals every day, with snacks as necessary in between. You can prevent feeling overly hungry and keep a constant blood sugar level by doing this.

Abstain from Strict Diets

Binge eating can also result from restrictive diets. You may experience intense desires when you deprive yourself of particular foods or dietary groups, which may cause you to overeat. Furthermore, restricted diets can be challenging to maintain over time, which can cause feelings of frustration and failure. Focus on eating a balanced diet that consists of a range of foods rather than adhering to a strict diet.

Discover Constructive Coping Strategies

Many people use food as a coping mechanism for painful emotions. To manage stress and anxiety, you can employ a variety of other healthy coping strategies. Exercise, meditation, deep breathing, and journaling are a few examples. Choose the coping skills that are most effective for you and incorporate them into your daily routine.

Get Expert Assistance

It's critical to get professional assistance if binge eating is a problem for you. A mental health expert can provide you with techniques for controlling your emotions and behaviors as well as help you discover the underlying problems that may be causing your binge eating. A licensed dietician can also assist you in creating a healthy eating strategy that satisfies your nutritional requirements.

However, it should be noted that preventing binge eating needs a mix of self-awareness, appropriate eating practices, and healthy coping mechanisms. You can keep a healthy connection with food and prevent binge eating by being aware of your triggers, engaging in mindful eating, eating regularly, avoiding restrictive diets, developing good coping skills, and getting professional assistance. Always remember to treat yourself nicely and ask for assistance if you need it.

Chapter 7

Strategies For Adaptation

Strategies For Adapting A Bodybuilding Meal Plan To Different Goals And Lifestyles, Such As Vegan Or Vegetarian Diets, Weight Loss Or Maintenance Goals, And Time-crunched Schedules

Bodybuilding is a demanding and rewarding activity that calls for a lot of commitment and effort. An effective food plan that supplies the nutrients required for muscle growth and recovery is an essential part of any successful bodybuilding regimen. But not everyone has the same dietary requirements or lifestyle. This session will provide tips on how to modify a bodybuilding meal plan to suit various dietary restrictions, time constraints, and lifestyles, such as vegan or vegetarian diets.

Vegetarian Or Vegan Diets

It's crucial to check that a person eating a vegan or vegetarian diet is still getting enough protein in their diet. Beans, lentils, tofu, and tempeh are just a few examples of plant-based foods that are rich in protein, which is necessary for both muscle growth and repair. Vegan protein supplements can also be used to increase protein intake.

It's crucial to pay attention to additional necessary minerals including iron, calcium, and vitamin B12. Spinach, lentils, and quinoa are examples of plant-based supplies of iron, whereas leafy greens, fortified plant-based milk, and tofu are sources of calcium. Supplements, fortified cereals, and nutritional yeast are all good sources of vitamin B12.

Objectives for Weight Loss or Maintenance

It's crucial to concentrate on portion control and calorie intake for people who want to lose weight or keep it off. Although modifications should be made to the portion sizes and overall calorie count, a bodybuilding meal plan can still be implemented.

Focusing on high-volume, low-calorie foods like fruits and vegetables is one tactic. These foods can help you feel full while also offering fiber and important nutrients. Also, cutting less on calorie-dense meals like sugary drinks and processed snacks can aid in lowering daily caloric intake.

Time-Constrained Calendars

Meal preparation and planning can be extremely helpful for people with busy schedules. Making meals ahead of time will help you make sure that you follow your meal plan and get the right nutrients throughout the day. To make meal planning and preparation easier, think about using slow cookers, instant pots, or meal prep services.

Another tactic for people with busy schedules is to concentrate on quick and simple food options. Pre-packaged protein drinks, bars, and ready-to-eat meals can be practical choices while still supplying vital nutrients for muscle development and recovery.

In conclusion, it's important to pay attention to unique dietary requirements, calorie consumption, and time management while modifying a bodybuilding meal plan to suit various goals and lifestyles. There are ways to make sure that your meal plan is supplying the nutrients you need for success in your bodybuilding endeavors, regardless of whether you are trying to lose weight, maintain your current weight, or have a hectic schedule. Always seek advice from a licensed dietician or other medical practitioners before making significant dietary changes.

Healthy And Delicious Meal Ideas For Vegetarian And Vegan Bodybuilders

A balanced and nourishing diet is necessary for bodybuilding to assist muscle growth and recuperation. It can be difficult for vegetarian and vegan bodybuilders to obtain the necessary amounts of protein and nutrients without using animal products. But, it is feasible to have scrumptious and healthful meals that complement bodybuilding objectives with a little imagination and organization. For vegetarian and vegan bodybuilders, I'll offer some tasty and nutritious food suggestions below.

Breakfast Bowl with Tofu Scramble

This breakfast bowl is brimming with protein and other necessary nutrients to get your day off to a healthy start. Start with quinoa or brown rice as a basis, then add sautéed vegetables like spinach, mushrooms, and onions. Then, scramble some tofu with your preferred flavors, including garlic powder, cumin, and turmeric. For a tasty and filling breakfast, add some avocado slices and a drizzle of spicy sauce on top.

Sweet Potato and Lentil Stew

This substantial stew's abundance of protein, fiber, and complex carbohydrates makes it the ideal post-workout meal. It is prepared by simmering sweet potatoes, lentils, diced tomatoes, onion, garlic, and your preferred seasonings in vegetable broth. For more flavor and nutrients, add some kale or other leafy greens toward the end of cooking.

Quinoa and Chickpea Salad

The small lunch or dinner that this salad makes is both filling and reviving. Cucumber, tomato, and bell pepper are simply mixed with cooked quinoa and chickpeas. Fresh herbs like parsley and cilantro can be added, and a straightforward vinaigrette composed of olive oil, lemon juice, and Dijon mustard can be used to season it.

Protein Smoothie for Vegans

Try a vegan protein smoothie for a quick and simple protein boost. For a tasty and nourishing beverage, blend frozen berries, bananas, plant-based milk, and your preferred vegan protein powder. For additional nutrients and fiber, you can also add some spinach or kale.

Black Bean Vegan Burgers

These flavorful burgers make the ideal post-workout meal or addition to a weekend barbecue. Mash cooked black beans with breadcrumbs, minced onion, minced garlic, and your preferred seasonings to make them. Make patties out of the mixture, then grill or bake them until crispy. Serve with toppings like avocado, tomato, and vegan cheese on a whole-grain bun.

Vegetarian and vegan bodybuilders have access to a wide variety of wholesome and delectable food options that can satisfy their vitamin and protein requirements. It is feasible to enjoy filling meals that support bodybuilding objectives by incorporating a mix of plant-based proteins, complete grains, and nutrient-dense vegetables. To make sure that your diet satisfies your individual needs, don't forget to see a licensed dietician or other medical specialists.

Sample Meal Plans For Different Bodybuilding Goals And Training Levels

A balanced and nourishing diet is necessary for bodybuilding to assist muscle growth and recuperation. You may maximize your nutrition and attain your desired outcomes by using a meal plan that is customized to your bodybuilding objectives and training level. Below are the illustrative meal plans for various bodybuilding objectives and levels of exercise. exercise

Food Plan for Novice Bodybuilders

If you are new to bodybuilding, your main objective should be to develop a solid nutritional basis and create appropriate eating practices. Whole, nutrient-dense foods that promote muscle growth and recovery should be the main focus of your meal plan. A sample menu for a novice bodybuilder is provided below:

1. Oatmeal with almond milk, a banana, and peanut butter for breakfast

2. Greek yogurt with berries and almonds as a snack

3. Lunch will be grilled chicken breast with mixed vegetables and sweet potatoes.

4. Apples and almond butter for a snack

5. The supper will be roasted Brussels sprouts and salmon with quinoa.

6. Protein shake with almond milk and banana as a post-workout snack

Food Plan for Intermediate Bodybuilders

After forming a healthy eating routine, you may concentrate on maximizing your nutrition for lean muscle growth and recuperation. With a focus on nutrient timing, your meal plan should have a balance of protein, carbohydrates, and healthy fats. An example food schedule for an intermediate bodybuilder is shown below:

1. Egg white omelet for breakfast with spinach, mushrooms, and avocado

2. Cottage cheese with berries and walnuts for a snack

3. Brown rice and a variety of veggies with grilled chicken or tofu for lunch.

4. Protein bar and fruit for a snack.

5. Steak or tempeh for supper with sweet potatoes and asparagus

6. Protein smoothie made with almond milk, banana, and oats as a post-workout snack.

Food Plan for an Advanced Bodybuilder

Your objective as an experienced bodybuilder is to maximize muscle growth and recovery through nutrition. A range of nutrient-dense meals should be included in your meal plan, with an emphasis on nutritional timing and supplementation. A sample menu for an advanced bodybuilder is provided below:

1. Greek yogurt and berries with protein pancakes for breakfast.

2. Beef jerky with almonds as a snack

3. Lunch would be quinoa, mixed vegetables, and grilled chicken or tempeh.

4. Protein smoothie made with almond milk and peanut butter for a snack.

5. The supper will be sweet potato and broccoli with bison or seitan.

6. Protein smoothie with almond milk, banana, oats, and creatine as a post-workout snack

Meal Plan For Vegetarian Bodybuilders

It can be difficult for vegetarian bodybuilders to obtain the necessary amounts of protein and nutrients without using animal products. But, it is feasible to have scrumptious and healthful meals that complement bodybuilding objectives with a little imagination and organization. A sample diet for a vegetarian bodybuilder is provided below:

1. Breakfast: Tofu scramble over whole grain toast with spinach and mushrooms

2. Greek yogurt with berries and almonds as a snack

3. Lunch: quinoa, mixed vegetables, and avocado in a chickpea salad.

4. Apples and almond butter for a snack

5. The supper will consist of lentil soup, sweet potatoes, and mixed greens.

6. Vegan protein smoothie with almond milk and banana as a post-workout snack

Bodybuilders of all levels need to have a balanced and nourishing diet. You may maximize your nutrition and attain your desired outcomes by customizing your food plan to your bodybuilding objectives and training level. To make sure that your diet satisfies your individual needs, don't forget to see a licensed dietician or other medical specialists.

Chapter 8

Meal Prep Hacks

Meal Prep Hacks For Busy Women

Many women are balancing various responsibilities in today's fast-paced society, including work, family, and social obligations. With so much to do, dinner preparation might frequently be put last on the list of things to accomplish. Meal preparation, however, is a crucial part of living a healthy and balanced lifestyle and can ultimately help you save time and money. For busy women, I'll offer food preparation Hacks in this chapter that will make it simple.

Schedule A Specific Time To Prepare Meals

Setting up a specific time each week for meal preparation is one of the secrets to effective meal preparation. This can take place for a few hours on a weekend day or a weeknight. You may make sure you have the time and energy to concentrate on meal preparation by arranging this time in advance.

Make A Meal Plan In Advance

Spend some time organizing your weekly meals before you start meal prep. This can speed up the meal preparation process and help you make sure you have all the necessary materials on hand. To help you keep organized and on schedule, think about using a meal planning tool or template.

Get High-quality Containers For Food Storage

Meal preparation can be significantly sped up and made easier by using high-quality food storage containers. Choose containers that are strong, impervious to leaks, and simple to stack and store. To accommodate various meals and servings, take into consideration purchasing containers in a range of sizes.

Make Use Of Kitchen Tools To Save Time

Numerous kitchen tools help speed up and simplify the food preparation process. Try purchasing a slow cooker or pressure cooker, which might make it easy for you to prepare meals in advance. You may also prepare ingredients fast by chopping vegetables in a food processor or using a mandoline slicer.

Cooking Basic Ingredients In Bulk

Rice, quinoa, and roasted veggies can all be batch cooked to save time and make meal preparation much simpler. These ingredients can be added to salads and bowls or used as a base for dinners throughout the week. They can also be quickly reheated.

Make Snacks Ahead Of Time

Making snacks ahead of time can prevent you from opting for bad options when you're hungry. Consider making snacks such as hard-boiled eggs, sliced vegetables with hummus, or homemade energy balls to have on hand throughout the week.

Use Leftovers

It's a terrific way to save time and reduce food waste to repurpose leftovers. Think about incorporating leftover grilled chicken or roasted vegetables in a salad or sandwich.

In summary, busy women don't necessarily need to be intimidated by meal preparation. You can make meal preparation simple and enjoy wholesome meals throughout the week by setting aside committed time, planning meals in advance, buying high-quality food storage containers, using kitchen tools, batch-cooking core items, making snacks ahead of time, and reusing leftovers.

Hacks On How To Meal Prep On A Tight Budget

A fantastic approach to saving time, eating well, and maintaining your fitness objectives is through meal planning. Yet it's simple to spend more than you should on groceries and meal prep supplies, which may rapidly mount up and strain your budget. The following are Hacks on how to meal prep on a tight budget so you may reap its rewards without going bankrupt.

Make A Meal Plan In Advance

Planning your meals in advance is one of the keys to meal preparation on a budget. Making a list of the ingredients you need will help you avoid overspending on food or buying needless goods. To help you keep organized and on schedule, think about using a meal planning tool or template.

Purchase Discounted And Seasonal Vegetables

Shopping for deals and produce that is in season is another method to cut costs on groceries. Plan your meals around the things that are on sale by looking through the weekly fliers of the grocery stores in your area. Consider including more seasonal fruits and vegetables in your meals since in-season produce is frequently less expensive and fresher than out-of-season produce.

Bulk Purchases

Additionally, buying in bulk might help you save money on groceries, particularly when purchasing common components like rice, quinoa, and dried beans. To save money per serving, think about buying these foods in bigger quantities from bulk bins or online sellers.

Cook In Groups

Batch cooking is a terrific way to cut costs and prep time for meals. Make a large batch of soup or chili that can be divided into portions and frozen for later use. Also, you can prepare a lot of chicken or ground beef and use it in various recipes all week.

Employ Reusable Containers For Meal Preparation

Since you won't need to buy throwaway containers regularly, investing in reusable meal prep containers can result in long-term financial savings. Look for containers that are strong, leak-proof, and simple to stack and store.

Use leftovers

A further technique to reduce the cost of meal preparation is to reuse leftovers. Think about incorporating leftover grilled chicken or roasted vegetables in a salad or sandwich. By incorporating leftovers into a wrap or quesadilla, you may create a brand-new dinner.

Make Food From Scratch

Making meals from scratch can help you spend less on processed and pre-packaged food. Make your sauces, dressings, and marinades because they can be cheaper and healthier than store-bought alternatives.

In summary, meal preparation on a tight budget is doable with a little forethought and imagination. You may reap the benefits of meal prep without going overboard on groceries by planning your meals in advance, searching for deals and in-season produce, buying in bulk, cooking in batches, using reusable meal prep containers, reusing leftovers, and cooking from scratch.

Time-saving Cooking Hacks And Ways To Maximize The Use Of Your Kitchen Appliances

The kitchen is frequently the center of the home, and many of us make it a habit to cook and prepare meals every day. But doing so can be a time-consuming and occasionally difficult undertaking. Thankfully, there are a variety of appliances and culinary techniques that can make the process quicker, simpler, and more fun. This session will discuss various time-saving cooking Hacks and ways to maximize the use of your kitchen appliances.

Quick Pot

A flexible kitchen appliance, the Instant Pot may be used for a variety of culinary techniques, including pressure cooking, slow cooking, and sautéing. You can prepare meals in a fraction of the time with an Instant Pot then you would without one. It is perfect for batch cooking and meal preparation because it is also wonderful for preparing huge quantities of food.

A Fryer

Making crispy, fried foods without using additional oil or calories is possible with the help of an air fryer. The dish is given a crispy outside and tender interior by hot air circulating it. It works well for preparing items like fish fillets, chicken wings, and French fries.

Food Processor

A food processor is a multipurpose appliance that can be used for chopping, slicing, shredding, and pureeing, among other things. It works well for chopping vegetables and nuts, as well as for preparing homemade sauces, dips, and salads.

Slow Cooker

A slow cooker is a fantastic appliance for quickly preparing meals. Simply throw your ingredients in the morning, and by the time supper rolls around, you'll have a delectable, slowly cooked meal. Stews, soups, and roasts cook beautifully in slow cookers.

Sheet Pan Dinners

Cooking an entire meal on a sheet pan requires little cleaning. Simply arrange your vegetables and protein on a baking sheet, season with your preferred seasonings, and roast in the oven. To make cleanup even simpler, you can also use aluminum foil or parchment paper.

One-Pot Dishes

One-pot meals are yet another excellent way to cut down on cooking time. All the ingredients for these meals are cooked in a single pot or skillet, which reduces cleanup and cooking time. Pasta dishes, casseroles, and stir-fries are a few examples of one-pot meals.

Pre-Cut and Pre-Washing Vegetables

For busy cooks, pre-cut and pre-washed vegetables can be a lifesaver. They work well as an ingredient in soups, salads, and stir-fries. They can also serve as the foundation for roasted veggies, which make for an easy and nutritious side dish.

In conclusion, there are a variety of appliances and time-saving cooking techniques that can make meal preparation and cooking simpler and more effective. You may spend less time and effort in the kitchen while still preparing great, healthy meals by using appliances like the Instant Pot, air fryer, food processor, and slow cooker as well as cooking methods like sheet pan meals and one-pot meals. Why not try out these suggestions and see if they can help you maximize your time in the kitchen?

Chapter 9

How To Maintain Your Motivation And Commitment To Your Meal Prep And Nutrition Goals

Meal planning and dietary compliance can be difficult, especially when life becomes hectic and other responsibilities start to take precedence. To achieve your nutrition and meal preparation goals and reach your health and fitness objectives, you must remain consistent. I will go over some advice for maintaining motivation and consistency with meal preparation and nutrition goals in this session.

Establish Attainable Objectives

Establishing attainable goals is essential for maintaining motivation and consistency.

Start with tiny, attainable goals that will help you gain momentum and confidence rather than creating a big aim that might be difficult to fulfill. You can gradually raise your targets as you reach these objectives.

Find a Supportive Network

When it comes to maintaining your motivation and consistency with your meal preparation and nutrition objectives, having a support system is crucial. Having someone to hold you accountable and provide support, whether it's a friend, a member of your family, or a personal trainer, can help you stay on track.

Simplicity Is Best

When meal prep and nutrition plans are overly complicated, they can be difficult to follow. By concentrating on full, nutrient-dense foods and avoiding processed foods, you can keep things simple. To save time and energy during the workweek, try batching your meal preparation.

Enjoy Your Success

Take some time to celebrate your victories when you accomplish a goal or move closer to your nutritional objectives. Celebrating your victories can keep you inspired and strengthen your dedication to your objectives.

Follow Your Development

Another excellent strategy to maintain motivation and consistency with your meal preparation and nutrition objectives is to keep track of your progress. Maintain a log of your diet, exercise, and advancement toward your objectives. Seeing your development on paper can keep you motivated and focused.

Don't Be Hard on Yourself

It can be difficult to follow a nutrition plan and prepare meals, and you could occasionally make mistakes or veer off course. It's crucial to avoid criticizing oneself when this occurs. Instead, accept what happened, take lessons from it, and continue.

Make It Entertaining

Nutritional regimens and meal preparation don't have to be monotonous or constricting. Consider integrating your favorite foods and recipes to make them more fun. Test out new dishes and play around with seasonings and ingredients.

Accomplishing your health and fitness goals requires keeping committed to your meal preparation and dietary objectives. You may maintain motivation and consistency with your meal preparation and nutrition objectives by making them enjoyable, setting achievable goals, enlisting support, keeping things simple, celebrating your victories, charting your progress, and not beating yourself up. You may reach your fitness and health goals over time, leading a healthier, happier life.

Conclusion

Success Stories And Interviews With Female Bodybuilders Who Used Proper Diet And Meal Preparation To Reach Their Goals

Many people who want to be physically active and healthy find inspiration in female bodybuilders. Dedication, effort, and a carefully thought-out nutrition plan are all necessary to develop the desired body. In this last part of the book, I'll share some energizing success stories and interviews with female bodybuilders who used meal planning and wise nutrition to attain their goals.

Karen McDougal

Bodybuilder, fitness model, and former Playboy Playmate Karen McDougal have won various fitness competitions. She is well renowned for her slim figure and has been in numerous magazines and TV shows. Karen credits a combination of exercise and wise eating for her accomplishment. She consumes a lot of protein and has small, regular meals throughout the day. She stresses the value of meal planning and preparation, saying that it keeps her on track and prevents temptation.

Dana Linn Bailey

Professional bodybuilder, businesswoman, and fitness icon Dana Linn Bailey. The Arnold Classic is just one of the bodybuilding competitions she has won. Nutrition, in Dana's opinion, forms the basis of a physically healthy and fit body. She consumes complex carbohydrates, lean protein, and good fats as part of a balanced diet. She stresses the significance of monitoring calories and macros as well as maintaining consistency in meal preparation and planning.

Ashley Kaltwasser

Professional bodybuilder and three-time Olympia champion Ashley Kaltwasser. She attributes her nutritional regimen, which emphasizes lean protein, complex carbohydrates, and healthy fats, to her success. During the off-season, she consumes fewer carbohydrates while increasing them during the preparation for competitions. Ashley stresses the value of meal planning and preparation, saying that it keeps her on track and prevents temptation.

Jamie Eason

Jamie Eason is a former NFL cheerleader, writer, and fitness model. She is renowned for her toned and slender physique and has won numerous fitness competitions. Jamie thinks that maintaining a healthy and fit body is all about nutrition. She consumes complex carbohydrates, lean protein, and good fats as part of a balanced diet. She stresses the value of meal planning and preparation, saying that it keeps her on track and prevents temptation.

Paige Hathaway

Fitness model and businesswoman Paige Hathaway is a multiple bodybuilding competition champion. She is renowned for her toned and slim body and has graced the covers of numerous magazines. Nutrition, in Paige's opinion, forms the basis of a physically healthy and fit body. She consumes complex carbohydrates, lean protein, and good fats as part of a balanced diet. She stresses the significance of monitoring calories and macros as well as maintaining consistency in meal preparation and planning.

In conclusion, many people who aim to be physically fit and healthy find inspiration in these female bodybuilders. Dedication, effort, and a carefully thought-out nutrition plan are all necessary to develop the desired body. Everyone may reach their fitness objectives by eating a balanced diet that contains lean protein, complex carbs, and healthy fats, tracking macronutrients and calories, and being consistent with meal planning and preparation. These triumph stories and interviews with female bodybuilders serve as a timely reminder that everything is attainable with effort, commitment, and wise dietary choices.

www.ingramcontent.com/pod-product-compliance
Lightning Source LLC
Chambersburg PA
CBHW070843250726
48662CB00003B/1333